HEALING YOURSELF

A Guide to Mind, Body, and Spirit Wellness | Reclaim
your health and happiness

By

ROLAND RICHARD

Disclaimer

This book has been written for informational purposes only. Every effort has been made to make this eBook as complete and accurate as possible. However, there may be mistakes in typography or content. Also, this e-book provides information only up to the publishing date. Therefore, this eBook should be used as a guide - not as the ultimate source.

The purpose of this eBook is to educate. The author and publisher do not warrant that the information contained in this e-book is fully complete and shall not be responsible for any errors or omissions.

The author and publisher shall have neither liability nor responsibility to any person or entity with respect to any loss or damage caused or alleged to be caused directly or indirectly by this e-book.

DEDICATION

This e-book is dedicated to every hurting person who has been through a lot in life, hoping to see the sunshine again and start having the desired impact.

You are not alone!

TABLE OF CONTENTS

Introduction

I'm so sick of all the bad vibes here! Do you? This world is unhealthy and polluted. I detest reading the newspaper, watching the news, and even talking to my neighbors. I don't want to seem like an outcast. I truly care about others. But this world has turned us into icy, ruthless people.

A society of dissatisfied individuals is the outcome. Divorce occurs in well over half of all marriages. Over half of all young individuals do not even think that marriage exists. We need to go back to the time when being nice was commonplace and it was easy to chat with strangers.

Those were the days when neighbors watched out for one another and people genuinely believed in love. We must recommit to loving ourselves. Every one of us must act to be the change we would like to see in the world. We must begin to mend and love ourselves once more.

Successful people are those who are joyful. This is due to the simple fact that happiness makes it easy to maintain motivation to accomplish your goals. Your perceptions have a huge influence on how you live your life and how well you get along with your loved ones, friends, and other people.

Even some claim that more than any other factor, our attitudes and beliefs can affect our health. Think about these instances:

- o A middle-aged man passes away a day after his doctor gave him a cancer diagnosis, despite the fact that an autopsy showed the doctor made a mistake.

- o Despite not being pregnant, many women who are desperate to have a baby start to exhibit real pregnancy symptoms, such as cravings and a growth in the size of their breasts.

- o Participants in clinical trials for new antidepressants who have depression start to feel better about themselves even if they were just given a placebo and not the genuine medication.

Having said that, it has been documented that changing the way you think about yourself and the world around you may significantly enhance your relationships, career, and health. This is considerably less expensive than hiring a divorce lawyer or paying for therapy sessions.

The goal of this book is to assist you in healing yourself of all the wounds and the effects of the surrounding negativity. I promise that if you learn to escape the suffering of this world, your overall health will significantly improve going forward.

Chapter 1: – Know Thyself

"The more you know yourself, the more patience you have for what you see in others." Erik Erikson

Knowing who you really are is a critical component of self-healing. If you are merely drifting through life without knowing who you are or what you won't stand for, how can you prevent a catastrophe?

There is a reason why an ambitious small-town girl who moves to the big metropolis frequently finds herself in a depressing and, dare I say, precarious scenario.

Consider the disgruntled Doctor as well, who is only a doctor because his parents insisted he be the first doctor in their family.

What about the mama's boy who is chosen at random and dates a girl he despises just to please his mother? These three have many characteristics.

Their issue can be explained by the proverb that states that if we don't know where we're going, any route will lead there. Even better, "if we do not stand for anything, we will fall for anything" is a good motto to live by. In other words, if we don't know who we are—our aims, dreams, and aspirations—anyone can easily influence us to make a choice that we'll regret for the rest of our lives.

Living with a decision you regret will be one of the hardest things you've ever had to do, especially if you have to deal with its repercussions every day. Living with the consequences of these decisions is a big factor in why so many individuals are so abrasive and cruel. I don't want you to live your life this way.

We will get the keys to unlocking our own potential when we take the time to comprehend who we truly are and the nuances of our own personalities. If you do not understand what it involves, you can also become your best self. You are often more likely to choose a career that you enjoy when you are aware of who you are.

And while you are building a career you are enthusiastic about, it is pretty simple to be driven with a passion to accomplish great things.

In addition, once you're at your best, you will look for the types of friends and relationships that will bring you joy and help you be your best self. They will be able to relate to your way of thinking and may even share it.

These are the people who won't mock your ambitions or be envious of your achievements. You'll become kinder, happier, and, dare I say it, more successful if you're surrounded by kind, helpful individuals.

People with a strong sense of self are frequently more determined and upbeat. Because they have complete control over the decisions they make regarding their lives, these people do well. Where others perceive obstacles, they are more inclined to recognize an opportunity.

Additionally, when you appreciate what you do, productivity comes much more easily.

Furthermore, the fact that you love your job will offer you an advantage over the competition, and you won't need other people's approval to motivate you. The joy of a sense of accomplishment will motivate you to keep going.

I am aware that these circumstances may appear ideal, where our decisions are not influenced by the wishes of our family and where we have been resilient enough to resist the pressure they will exert on us to choose a particular option.

But trust me when I say that getting to know and fully understanding yourself will provide you access to chances you would not otherwise have seen coming.

When you are certain of the choice that is best for you, it will be easier for you to resist the pressure from those around you. I'm not telling you to ignore your obligations to support your family; rather, I'm telling you to know who you really are and to always be true to your identity. When you are not living with the burden of a wrong decision for the long term, you will be much more joyful and easier to love.

How to Discover Yourself

Even if it's easier said than done, it's not impossible. Start by conducting some impartial analysis. This does not entail merely asking others in your immediate vicinity what they think of you.

Negative or positive encounters you have with them will stop them from being as impartial as you require. Using a credible personality test is a preferable choice. The Myers-Briggs- specific personality test is a well-liked choice.

Which of the 16 personality types described by this theory best describes you will be determined by this test. It has grown in popularity recently because you can use the results to find out what kind of setting you work best in and even how you connect with other people.

In addition, whether you choose the outcomes or not, they frequently exhibit astonishing accuracy.

Another excellent choice is exams of career aptitude. These are made to make it easier for someone like you to comprehend your skill set and how you may use it to choose the best vocation. You can pursue a career that you love at any time.

Until you have a well-thought-out plan in place that will enable you to take care of your obligations while also pursuing a passion project, go for it.

Money may be limited, and you may already be pressed for time, making it unlikely that you can act at this moment. However, I would advise you to keep getting ready. Continue picking up as much information as you can about that profession online or from those around you.

This will put you in a position to seize an opportunity if it presents itself.

When you take the time to get to know yourself, you can uncover some unfinished business and hidden traumas that you likely would have preferred to keep buried.

Regrettably, you have been displaying these scars in your interactions with others every day. You might have become too soft or just too indifferent to care about other people's feelings as a result of these wounds.

Become the absolute best version of yourself now that you can see yourself clearly. Respect yourself. Above all, always be true to who you are. Knowing your limitations is yet another critical ability to develop in order to survive on this chaotic planet. The following chapter will cover this.

Chapter 2: Know Your Limits

"A great man is always willing to be little." — *Ralph Waldo Emerson*

The portion that lists your strengths and weaknesses is an important component of the Myers-Briggs Personality type test results.

If we had been a little more aware of our limitations, many of the mistakes and issues we run into may have been completely avoided. Just picture a weightlifter who is overly eager and attempts to lift too much too quickly.

What do you anticipate happening? Any sensible individual will understand that the weightlifter will end up hurting themselves. Some will claim that this example promotes self-limitation, and if we do that and stop challenging ourselves, we will never realize our actual potential.

If you put your mind to anything, there are no limits to what you can accomplish, and sometimes you won't know how powerful we really are until you try.

To attain your objectives, you must, however, make sure that a workout today with 20 pounds could be a better option if you've never lifted 100 pounds. There really is nothing improper with having a big-picture approach, but

I would advise starting small and working your way up. In essence, I'm telling you to have reasonable expectations. Being modest will not only prevent you from having lofty aspirations, but it will also enable you to set reasonable deadlines for completing your tasks.

A lot of individuals become frustrated when they are certain they haven't accomplished a particular objective. But simply think about how different Mark Zuckerberg is from Colonel Sanders.

Colonel Sanders didn't start Kentucky Fried Chicken (KFC) until after he was 80 years old, whereas Mark Zuckerberg started his Facebook corporation in his early 20s. Although both men are regarded as being tremendously successful, their success came at various times.

Perhaps you are simply not in the correct industry, or it is simply not the proper time for you. Finding a career in a sector you are passionate about will help you maintain inspiration and achieve success, as was discussed in Chapter 1. The lives of these two guys provide evidence for this theory. Their zeal for what they loved led to their achievement.

You can avoid comparing your accomplishments to those of others by living a modest lifestyle. Some struggle to climb the ladder, while others strike the ball out of the park on their first attempt.

Some people get married as soon as they graduate from college, while others must wait a while and kiss a few frogs before they locate the proper match. In actuality, both Mark Zuckerberg and Colonel Sanders faced numerous obstacles on their own paths to success. And so will you. Do not contemplate a difference in your world. No matter what you want to accomplish, you will have to put in more effort than you ever have and perhaps wait a bit longer than you anticipated.

Being modest has many attractive features that go well beyond accomplishment. This trait will prevent you from trying to chew off far more than you can handle. Not every request needs to be accepted. This holds true for both your personal and professional lives.

If you really want to impress your employer, don't accept deadlines that are too tight unless you are quite certain you can meet them. If you don't know how to complete an assignment that you've been given, do not be reluctant to seek assistance.

Don't overcommit at your child's school if you have a family to support and a full-time job to attend to. Know your limits. This holds true for your time, effort, feelings, and abilities. The very next chapter will explain how modesty equates with honesty and how you may use it to better your life and heal yourself.

Chapter 3: – Be Honest

"Honesty is the fastest way to prevent a mistake from turning into a failure." James Altucher

A thief seems to be the only thing worse than a liar. Liars make life challenging and are frequently unaware of the extensive consequences of their conduct.

Lying makes us miserable people because we have to continuously watch our backs and cover our records. In actuality, few things are as poisonous as a liar.

Never should we let the negative in this world drive us to deceive others. Your proximity to the cheating and stealing door will increase if you lie. Stop now while you're ahead. Just consider the potential results of one dishonest act:

- Loss of income

- Loss of self-respect;

- ▢ Permanent harm to another person's reputation

- ▢ Permanent harm to relationships

- ▢ Permanent harm to your reputation

- ▢ Guilty feelings

- ▢ Sleep loss

- ▢ Diminished trust

The words respect, truthfulness, impartiality, integrity, uprightness, virtue, and truthfulness can all be used as synonyms for the word honesty. It takes more than just not lying when things are tough, to be honest.

Being morally straight in all circumstances is a requirement for honesty. In other words, we shall make every effort to be truthful and regain the trust of those around us through our deeds. But being honest can be very tough. It is challenging to enumerate every situation where honesty is required.

18

If you're confused about whether anything you did was honest or not, a good test is whether you had to conceal it or trick someone into thinking you did something else.

You are probably not being honest if you feel the need to cover your tracks after doing or saying something.

Any difficulties you may have as a consequence of this training pale in comparison to the advantages of being honest. Imagine the peace of mind it would provide you to not have to second-guess everything you do or continuously look over your shoulder for signs that you are being discovered.

Imagine not having the heaviness of guilt when you wake up as a result of what you did. And don't imagine that being honest serves no one's interests. Being drawn to and respecting an honest person is pretty simple. When looking for new employees or contemplating a potential promotion within their company, the majority of employers place the most importance on that quality.

Being truthful does not entail disclosing all of our private matters to everyone attempting to eavesdrop on our affairs. Instead, we really shouldn't withhold important information from people who are entitled to an honest response.

Avoiding the numerous strategies that will surface to obtain more now than we merit or trick others into thinking untrue things about us also involves being honest. However, there are instances when some of us could find ourselves in really disastrous situations as a result of being perceived as being quite honest.

When our remarks are not balanced with kindness, this is frequently the case. We'll look at how that quality can prevent many of the issues that can arise from that kind of communication in the following chapter.

Chapter 4: – Be Kind

"Kindness is the language that the deaf can hear and the blind can see." Mark Twain

Being nice entails being hospitable, thoughtful, compassionate, and friendly. You need to be a friend in order to make one. The proverb "birds of a feather flock together" is even more overused. You have to be the kind of person who attracts joyful, encouraging individuals into your life. If not, why would anyone want to be around you?

People would remember how they felt as a result of an interaction for a very long time, as the astute Maya Angelou pointed out. When we act cruelly, we make life much tougher than it needs to be for others around us. When we are nasty or unfriendly, we make people feel unloved, undervalued, and alone.

Would you want that to happen to you? Would you appreciate being treated so harshly? Do you not believe that approaching people in that way at work, school, or even in your own home makes your life far more difficult than it needs to be? Even when people don't know each other well, kindness encourages cooperation.

It is far simpler to take on the world with the help of others than it is to try to do it on your own. Being unkind encompasses a wide range of behaviors. The most prevalent way we act rudely is through our words. Being unfriendly can be seen as being rude, condescending, or even abrupt.

It's not just rude to use words to disparage others and extol yourself; furthermore, it is a profoundly selfish action that frequently does more damage than good. Being polite is a crucial component of kindness. Let's spend some time getting to know this lovely quality better.

Why Be Polite and respectful?

It's not as difficult as some people are making it out to be. Because of the unkind attitudes of those around us, it is undeniable that being and courteous is getting harder, yet it is still achievable. These people's egos may be inflated by our politeness, but it does not reflect poorly on them.

Whatever the circumstance, being polite reflects favourably on our character. People who are courteous are frequently regarded as being nice, upright, competent, and pleasant. And in our highly linked society, it's impossible to tell who you could have offended.

Imagine how humiliated you would feel if you attended a job interview only to learn that the man you had just yelled at in the parking lot for parking in "your" place was actually the interviewer. You may experience it; believe me, it has occurred many times before.

Respecting and taking into account the needs, feelings, time, resources, values, and cultural conventions of others is part of being courteous. Being kind will make you very likeable and inspire others to show you the same courtesy. Being courteous will also make it quite simple for you to win the respect of others around you.

They will be made to regard you and your values even if they really do not immediately alter their behavior. They might eventually result in an improvement of your efforts.

If we all had employment where our coworkers, employees, and subordinates treated us with respect, wouldn't life be a lot simpler? Being nice is one of the simplest ways to garner respect, which must be earned.

Rules for Courtesy and Kindness

1. Don't say, post, or even think anything unkind if you don't have anything kind to say about it. Even whispered remarks to a buddy have been known to come back to bite the speaker.

2. Be generous with your salutations and greetings. If you walk into a room, give everyone a warm welcome. Please excuse yourself as you depart. And if someone greets you, give them a nice grin in return.

3. Don't belittle other people's efforts, especially when it's clear that they

worked hard to complete a task. If you must, follow up on any constructive criticism with an actual compliment.

4. Show gratitude for other people's efforts. There is no need to express your disapproval if what is offered doesn't suit you.

5. Try to gain some insight into the cultural mores and viewpoints of those who are close to you. You merely need to be informed enough to avoid unintentionally offending someone; you do not have to agree with their viewpoints.

   Allowing them to freely voice these opinions without worrying about being disrespected is also the polite thing to do. You can always come to an understanding.

6. You don't have to always demand that things be done your way. Every once in a while, let someone else shine.

7. Avoid dominating conversations by talking exclusively about yourself and your

achievements. Asking about oneself and paying attention to what they have to say demonstrates a genuine interest in the other person.

8. Pay close attention to what others are saying when they are speaking to you. Make eye contact and stop moving or typing or doing anything else.

When someone interrupts you gently because you are busy, take a moment to consider how long the conversation should last, let them know you value what they have to say, and then set up a more convenient time to continue.

Chapter 5: – Be Forgiving

"The weak can never forgive. Forgiveness is the attribute of the strong." - Gandhi

Forgiveness is not always simple. The simple fact that we have to use the word suggests that we have suffered some sort of harm. One of the biggest presents you can offer yourself is to forgive a grudge, whether it is genuine or imagined.

Whether or not you think the person deserves such kindness, this is true. We develop resentment when we resist forgiveness. It's like drinking poison and expecting the person who hurt us to perish when we hold onto resentment. It's comparable to causing injuries to our own bodies and expecting someone else to experience the anguish.

This reasoning is not just flawed but also highly perilous. Hatred is an extremely unpleasant emotion that resentment can easily turn into.

But why is it so difficult for us to forgive? Why does the thought of letting go of the pain make us feel so uneasy if forgiving someone who has injured us can be so beneficial?

The actual issue is that none of us want to keep going through the agony of whatever evil was done to us. However, when we continue to reflect on how much we were harmed, we unintentionally start to consider holding the offender accountable.

Frequently, our misguided sense of fairness leads us to think that we will receive the justice we deserve if we cling onto every bit of the suffering that was inflicted and refuse to let it go.

This is especially true if the offender doesn't seem to regret their actions. Unfortunately, refusing them our friendship or goodwill out of resentment will not make the person change for the better. By forcing our minds to repeatedly experience the agony, we are just doing ourselves harm.

Our appearance, our words, and our attitude will all suffer as a result of the heavy weight of resentment that weighs heavily on our emotions as we storm violently through life.

Even if we could have just been harmed by one or a few people, everyone around us will start to feel the effects. We are frequently agitated, depressed, and otherwise highly unpleasant when we are resentful.

And to make matters worse, the people who suffer as a result of what happened are frequently the people we love rather than the ones who offended us.

Additionally, it has been shown that the burden of resentment has an impact on our recollection, performance at work, capacity for everyday chores, ability to concentrate, and even our desire for sex.

Immune system deterioration, poor cardiovascular health, and even increased blood pressure have all been connected to being resentful and reluctant to forgive. As you can see, failing to pardon others will never prove healthy.

But what exactly is forgiveness? Is it merely the forgetting of what happened? Does accepting forgiveness entail acting as if nothing happened? Nope. It's not that easy. When we pardon, we must go beyond just saying it.

We need to alter our attitudes toward the person. It seems as though we are giving them a fresh start from scratch. You are not going to stand by while the circumstances harm you or the other parties involved.

High emotional intelligence, self-control, and love are needed for this. Not only does forgiveness "get them off the hook" for what they did, but it also frees the individuals involved to put the past behind them and focus on the present.

"Forgiveness means that you fill yourself with love, and you radiate that love outward. You need to refuse to hang onto the venom or hatred that

was engendered by the behaviors that caused the wounds." Wayne Dye.

Giving someone the power to control your happiness by allowing yourself to become furious in response to their acts and to dwell on what happened for a protracted length of time It feels as though you are letting them control you, and they will keep doing so until you find the strength to forgive them.

Another reason forgiveness is advantageous is because it frequently follows self-awareness. When we keep in mind that we too have frequently had to seek forgiveness, forgiving others becomes simpler for us.

Despite what we might think, we really aren't perfect. Sometimes, without even realizing it, we injure those around us—even the ones we love. It will be easy for those close to us to forgive us when we make mistakes if we choose not to hold grudges and actively seek forgiveness. By simply being generous, we can all become much happier and more successful people in this world.

Several benefits of forgiving others include the following:

- o You'll feel considerably better and be much happier.

- o You won't put your job in danger by being unproductive.

- o You won't put your relationship with your significant other or your family in danger.

- o You'll get better sleep at night.

- o You'll gain more self-control and self-awareness, experience more peace, and earn the respect of those around you.

- o You won't feel as bad about the harm that was done

- o Your anxiety will decrease. As you become more conscious of your own inner strength, your self-esteem will rise.

What an absence of Forgiveness Is!

To be forgiving does not require you to be a pushover who continually allows themselves to be wounded.

While you will absolutely let go of whatever resentment you may have toward the offending party or parties, you should not have to put yourself in a position where you could experience the same type of harm.

After seeing what these people are capable of, it is totally reasonable to exercise a bit more caution. But please proceed with caution. Don't fall into the trap of believing that a person's actions speak for who they are when they commit minor infractions, which are ones that weren't done with malice aforethought. Please keep in mind that we are all humans and have all hurt someone.

Retaliation is not a possibility after forgiveness. It is not a declaration that you now have the "overwhelming advantage" to say you have forgiven someone. Even though the involved parties may have been at fault, they have no obligation to you.

By making this peace offering and letting go of the anger that formerly engulfed you, you have gained a lot, even if they do not apologize. Keep in mind that by being forgiving, you are benefiting yourself. Although they might gain from your choice, you are actually offering yourself a gift by forgiving them.

Tips for Forgiving

I would never expect that you would forgive someone who has wronged you instantly or all at once since we both know that doing so is difficult. You have the choice to provide forgiveness gradually.

By gradually letting go of your animosity toward those who have harmed you, you will give yourself enough time to purge all traces of your bitterness from your mind and heart. If you get the opportunity to visit this person often, you can start by just saying hello.

They may be surprised by this since they did not anticipate such a thoughtful act, and that can pave the way for the conversation you two need to have to reach a resolution. It is often preferable to make the effort to make things right, even when you have been wronged.

Regardless of whether they appreciate the gesture or not, always keep in mind how this modest action will benefit you in the long term.

Writing down the name of the person or people who hurt you and making a list of everything they have ever done to irritate you is another easy exercise that will enable us to forgive.

Once you've finished making that list, make a list of any of the times you've hurt someone and been forced to beg for their pardon. We don't usually think about things like this.

Having a clear understanding of how frequently we have caused harm to individuals close to us, especially to all those we love, may be the motivation we need to forgive.

Some people find it even more unsettling to read the list of people they dislike on the list of people they have had to seek forgiveness from.

Making a list of all the nice things this individual has done for you would be another fruitful exercise.

This activity can help you keep in mind that, in spite of their flaws, this person or those people also possess many lovely traits. These characteristics, in the case of the people closest to us, are the same reasons we loved them and initially held them close.

Just consider: by offering an olive branch of peace, you might be able to persuade that individual to see the error of their ways and make a positive change. If you had even helped one person improve their character, the world would be a better place. Such generosity is not unappreciated or unrewarded.

To be forgiving, one must be very resilient. But consider how much better our lives would be if we did not go through each day carrying bitterness and resentment. One of the best ways to cure ourselves is to release that oppressive burden. This planet is already in a terrible state, and increasing animosity would only make matters worse. The following chapter will detail how.

Chapter 6: – Be Generous

"If you can't feed a hundred people, then just feed one."—Mother Teresa

It is not necessary for a generous person to give away everything they own. A charitable person is also not compelled to put up with being used as a punching bag. First and foremost, being generous means being inclined to share more than is necessary or being ready to give.

Generosity elevates kindness to a new level. Even though you have a good heart and frequently consider ways to help others, you have not completely mastered the art of generosity until you take the initiative to start volunteering your time, effort, or other resources for the greater good of others. We are motivated by generosity to give of ourselves voluntarily without expecting anything in return.

I understand that you might be wondering how donating your assets will improve your quality of life. The truth is that the majority of people think that being generous is one of the secrets

38

to finding true happiness in this wretched world. Actually, a lot of doctors will testify that being kind is excellent for your health. In fact, the following are some definite advantages of generous giving:

- o Less stress

- o Lower risk of developing depression

- o Stronger sense of purpose

- o Greater happiness

- o better marriages and families

- o Reduced risk of dementia

- o Less clutter

- o Greater appreciation for what you already have

- o Higher likelihood of benefiting from others' giving

A generous individual frequently looks for opportunities to help others. Consider the volunteers who travel to soup kitchens every day to provide a meal. Those of us who have the courage to join the Peace Corps are also thought to be pretty kind.

However, even a small act of generosity, such as pausing to let a youngster cross the street or helping an old woman with her grocery bags, might be regarded as kind.

This kind of care for others is advantageous because it compels us to concentrate on their needs rather than our own issues. Anything that lessens the impact of our issues, whether they be interpersonal or financial, will have an immediate impact on our health.

Being generous shields us from the cynicism and vanity that make navigating this planet so complex.

However, I would advise you to use caution as you try to be more generous. Pay close attention to how you show others your kindness. Please exercise extra caution when giving to those of the opposing sex.

If you're already in a relationship and don't want to give the wrong impression, stay away from favours or presents that are too intimate. Anything involving one's body is considered a personal gift. For instance, perfume would be regarded as a personal present.

Please keep in mind that being generous may compromise your personal safety. When asked for money by a person who appeared to be homeless, many people have been robbed.

No matter how desperate the person seems to be, it's never a good idea to reach into your wallet or bag and show where and how much cash you have. Telling the person you'll be back with a gift is a safer course of action.

I would strongly advise that you pack up the stuff that you would like to present to this person in advance and go to a safe place that is away from inquisitive eyes.

The last bit of advice I have is to be cautious before being overly kind. Some individuals enjoy spontaneity, while others would rather you first inquire whether they need your assistance. Even the finest intentions can get you into awkward situations if they are not carried out properly.

We've talked at length about how developing different facets of your personality can aid in your self-healing and prevent you from carrying around a lot of the emotional problems that come with pessimism in this world. The most crucial key to removing all the scars left by this cruel world can be found in this book's conclusion. Please continue reading to find out more about that.

Chapter 7: – Be Yourself

"Be yourself; everyone else is already taken." — Oscar Wilde
"The greatest gift you ever give is your honest self." Fred Rogers

We all need to rediscover who we are. This is one of the most important components of surviving this tragedy we call life. This support does not in any way grant you license to do badly.

We've already talked about how we must work hard to overcome our unfavourable characteristics in order to be able to cure ourselves of the suffering this world has created.

Character flaws like haughtiness, rudeness, arrogance, and stinginess have no place in your life. We open the door to all kinds of negativity when we proudly carry out these repulsive behaviours. That simply leads to greater suffering and disappointment.

That is why I advised you to get to know yourself in the first chapter. By knowing more about your shortcomings, you will be better equipped to heal yourself.

So what does it mean to be yourself? You must remove yourself from all the tags that the people around you have placed on you. These demeaning labels are a result of the way we appear, how we dress, or even the neighbourhood where we were raised.

We have no justification for allowing the environment to shape us into a kind that doesn't accurately reflect who we are. Imagine how wonderful it would be to not have to put on a false persona. Of course, everything here is reasonable.

We wouldn't want to take some liberties that might have a significant impact on our personal lives and perhaps put our employment in danger. Consequently, you might just want to wait before making any major decisions, such as dyeing your hair green and emerald, until you find a job that will allow you to make such a decision.

Here are the top 5 reasons you should start living authentically:

1. It is impossible to win over everyone. If you constantly let the people around you define who you are, you'll constantly need to modify your values to appease everyone. Additionally, you won't be content with the results if you put yourself under that much strain.

2. The civilization that surrounds us is genuinely apathetic. Both the submissive housewife and the tenacious achiever are portrayed in the media as perfect women.

   Men must also be considerate of the requirements of the other sex as well as the dangerous bad boy, according to society. Which one will you be if you just let those around you define who you are? Whatever you want to be, keep in mind that putting up this kind of show every day is quite taxing.

3. You'll wind up making crucial decisions for your life depending on the whims of others close to you, who won't have to deal with the results.

   You will be the one who has to take care of the child if you decide to have one just because your family feels it's time! If you choose a career because your friends and family think you'll succeed in it, you'll be stuck with it for the rest of your life.

4. The reality always shines through. People will eventually figure out that you are lying. Unfortunately, the truth frequently comes out in a significant scandal or collapse, as we witness in the cases of many celebrities.

5. You will be genuinely happy when you are satisfied with who you are. When you are continuously trying to be someone you are not, how can you ever love yourself?

All things considered, if you really want to enjoy true progress, you must assume control over your life. If you are not courageous enough to make significant changes, you cannot predict different outcomes. And the moment has come for such changes!

Conclusion

I hope this book has been useful to you. I hope you have decided to make some much-needed improvements as a result of the benefit.

Although progress could be gradual at first, you won't ever regret choosing to better yourself. Every action, no matter how tiny, counts as progress because it moves us closer to our goals.

The good in us is rewarded by the universe, and it also assists us in seeing the good in others.

You should be aware by this point that we hold the key to our own recovery and to surviving the disaster that is life.

Our lives won't get any better unless we accept the mistakes we've made and actively work to fix them.

"As human beings, our greatness lies not so much in being able to remake the world—that is the myth of the atomic age—as in being able to remake ourselves." — Mahatma Gandhi